American

Physicians dedic

MW01592974

Physician-Patient Relations

Henrie Moise

A Guide to Improving Satisfaction

Physician-Patient Relations
A Guide to Improving Satisfaction

© 1999 by the American Medical Association

Printed in the USA.

All rights reserved.

Additional copies of this book may be ordered by calling toll free 800 621-8335.

Internet address: http://www./ama-assn.org

ISBN 0-89970-981-8

OP208699

BP5240:98-1157:2.5M:4/99

Acknowledgments

The author of this book is Henrie Moise, a Chicago-based writer. The following people also made significant contributions to this book. Their efforts are both acknowledged and appreciated.

Suzanne Fraker
Director
Product Line Development
Book and Product Group
American Medical Association

Karla Powell
Senior Editor
Product Line Development
Book and Product Group
American Medical Association

Michael Weitz
Manager, Marketing and Promotions
Sales and Marketing
Book and Product Group
American Medical Association

Selby Toporek
Senior Communications Coordinator
Marketing Services
Book and Product Group
American Medical Association

Michelle Ryan Bartlett
Image Coordinator
Marketing Services
Book and Product Group
American Medical Association

Contents

Introduction

Computer specialists coined the term "user friendly" in the late 1970s to designate systems designed to meet the public's needs. Substitute the word patient for "user" and that is what this book is all about. Much of what makes a service user-friendly is effective communication and efficient interaction. In recognizing the importance of these skills among physicians, their staff, as well as the patients themselves, the result is improved medical services.

Providing medical care that is accessible, convenient, and practiced in a "patient-friendly" manner will ultimately relieve physicians of many of the management burdens that can interfere with clinical responsibilities.

The demand for better health care systems is certain to accelerate as we enter the 21st century. The time is now to enhance satisfaction through optimal physician-patient relations.

Section 1

Understanding the Physician-Patient Relationship

Issues and Challenges

There's no doubt about it—"the times they are a changing," as the popular song goes. That's apparent almost everywhere you look, including right in your own practice. It's a common complaint among physicians that "patients just aren't what they used to be." And—if you were privy to the complaints of patients—you'd know soon enough that they think "doctors just aren't what they used to be."

Who can really blame either side? Patients no longer have health insurance that allows them unlimited choice of doctors and hospitals; and the days of fee-for-service practice for physicians are numbered, if not over. Yet despite these changes, the essence of medicine remains the same—*physicians entrusted to care for their patients.*

A good doctor-patient relationship can no longer be assumed. The demands of insurance companies, managed care organizations, government agencies, and other aspects of modern medicine require more effort today—by both parties. Yet even within these confines, it helps to keep the following in mind:

- Physicians *can* improve their relationships with patients.
- Patients will continue to select their physician—often based exclusively on the kind of relationship that exists.
- Physicians will have to take the lead in educating their patients about what, exactly, constitutes "appropriate" care.
- Together, patients and physicians can explore a wide range of options for health care services.

The patient/physician relationship is often affected by the *setting*. In hospitals, for instance, physicians are surrounded by medical specialists, therapists, nurses, technologists, pharmacists, social service professionals and others. These myriad people may intimidate patients; and in response they expect their physician to be friend and advocate, as well as healer.

In the doctor's office, things are somewhat less threatening. Yet even there, depending on size, physician assistants, nurses, technicians, receptionists, and billing personnel may (in their role as gatekeepers) stand between doctors and patients

As a result, patients are becoming more proactive about their health and treatment. With the Internet they now can get copious amounts of health information. Therefore, they may feel better prepared to participate in medical decision-making.

Improving patient-physician relations requires a two-sided effort since they enter this relationship with different expectations. It's worth it, though. A good relationship will ultimately result in better care and prove satisfying to both physicians and patients.

According to the Pfizer Medical Humanities Initiative survey of the patient-physician relationship in America, the most important things a doctor can do to develop a positive relationship—from the *patient's* perspective—are:

- Provide fast and efficient medical treatment.
- Establish a friendly rapport.
- Show compassion.

Doctors, on the other hand, say the most important things patients can do to develop a positive relationship are:

- Be open, honest, and thorough.
- Take an active interest in their own health—beyond simply following the physician's medical advice for a given problem.
- Keep track of the medications they are taking.

There are valuable insights to be gleaned from these two perspectives. Although they differ widely, each side can easily understand the other. None of these expectations is especially difficult to achieve, once they are spelled out in clear and simple terms.

For example, self-confident and assertive patients demand autonomy *and* highly personalized care. Such patients tend to seek a doctor who is humane, understanding, articulate, and accessible. If the physician seeks status in the relationship—such as trying to impress the patient with his or her knowledge of medicine and technology rather than sharing it—then trouble lies ahead.

When both physician and patient focus on the relationship, both tend to experience long-lasting satisfaction. Research shows that patient satisfaction leads to patient retention. It also indicates that when patient satisfaction exists, there are fewer malpractice claims. With managed care growing more concerned with such issues, the physician-patient relationship takes on added significance.

The Patient

The most significant demographic development in the past century has been the population's age distribution. Richard K. Thomas reports in his book, *Health Care Consumers in the 1990s*, that the elderly account for 40 to 50 percent of physician office visits. He continues, "The huge baby-boom generation is now entering its late 40s. Although the health conditions of aging begin to accumulate after age 45, the age at which the demand for health care services escalates has steadily risen. That means it will be another 20 years before the heaviest pressure will be felt within the health care system."

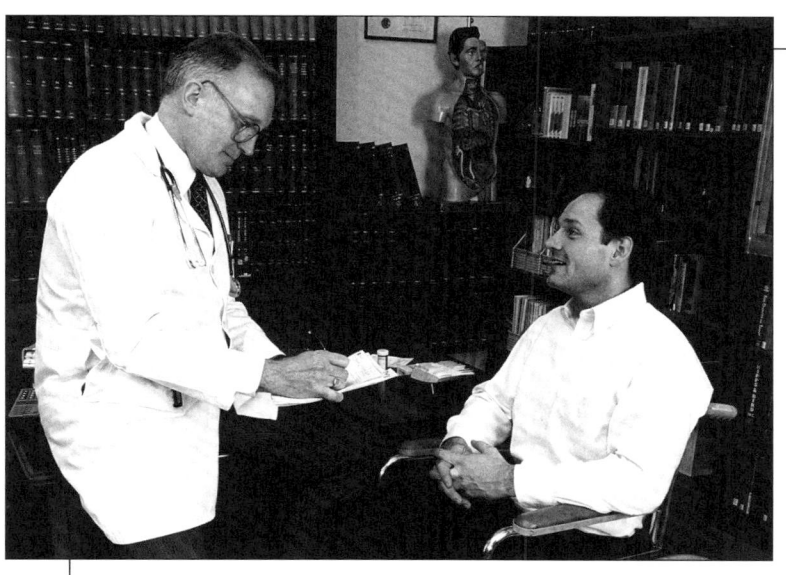

With more girls born today than boys and women living longer than men, "The significance of the 'feminization' of American society cannot be overstated," says Thomas. "Today, for example, more than 25 million women now head their own households. Women account for 60 percent of single-person households and 86 percent of single-parent households." Women make most of the decisions about use of health care services for themselves, their husbands and their families. In the case of the elderly, daughters are more likely to become caretakers and make the necessary medical decisions concerning their parents' health.

Another demographic factor is the generation to which a patient belongs. Patients who came of age during the Great Depression typically establish lasting relationships with their doctors whom, to them, "reign supreme." As a rule they follow doctor's orders and respect an approach to health care that consists of technology, treatment and cure.

Their children, born after World War II, are the "baby boomer" generation that "questions authority"—and the health care system is no exception. Many patients from this generation do not have an ongoing relationship with a particular doctor but instead favor the use of emergency rooms, ambulatory centers and freestanding clinics for their health care needs. They smoke less, drink in moderation, and have healthier diets. They are keenly interested in the prevention of disease and, if they do become ill, want to be a part of the healing process.

These baby boomers even have an influence on their elders in shaping a patient philosophy. If illness strikes their parents, they are on hand to question the doctor; and if hospitalization is required, they question hospital procedures as well. In turn, more and more parents are following their children's lead and becoming self-assertive and proactive about health matters.

Yet, regardless of generation:

- Every patient reacts to illness individually.
- Each is influenced by past experiences with hospitals and doctors. (Indeed, many put off going to a doctor for this reason.)
- They rely primarily on family and friends for recommendations about doctors and hospitals.
- They may have unrealistic expectations about treatment outcomes.
- Most patients are barraged with health care reports from television, newspapers, and magazines, and they don't know who or what to believe.

The Role of Families

The most obvious function the family plays for physicians is in helping them identify, prevent, or treat medical conditions through a thorough family history. A knowledge of family dynamics also may help explain various emotional illnesses and anxieties.

Yet because family is typically the patient's primary support system, medical professionals also must recognize the role it can play in facilitating the healing process. Involvement of family members in the treatment program can help achieve a positive outcome for both patient and physician.

An article in the June 1996 issue of the *Journal of Family Practice* reports on a study of family involvement in routine health care. This survey of patient behavior and preferences concludes that patients prefer more direct family involvement in their health care than what typically occurs. However, there is a wide discrepancy between patients who want family members or friends present during routine health care and those who want them present only if there are health problems. If physicians want to address these preferences, they might do so when taking a patient's medical history. At that time they can inquire whether the patient wants others involved in their health care and under what circumstances.

Patients' Point of View

Research has identified specific obstacles to a good physician-patient relationship. Are any of these found in your practice?

- **Red tape.** This frustration begins before the patient even sees a doctor. For example, maybe they had to undergo an elaborate referral process. Then, once they arrive for their appointment, they are faced with an onslaught of forms to sign, sometimes including a financial responsibility waiver.

- **Practice structure.** Many physicians who were solo practitioners have turned toward group practice or networks. While these new arrangements have many benefits for patients and physicians alike, patients sense decreased personal attention and closeness with their doctor.

- **Scheduling delays.** Patients may feel neglected if they are left seated in the reception area for long periods of time without any feedback from the receptionist as to whether the doctor is running late. Then, if the delay continues once they're ushered into the examination room, frustration may brew unnecessarily. Once the doctor appears, he or she often seems to be on a fast running clock. As a result, patient questions may go unasked; and the doctor himself may hurry important explanations and instructions.

- **Emergencies.** Trying to reach a doctor by telephone can be extremely frustrating for patients, especially in an emergency. They may face busy signals, long periods on "hold," and lost or misconstrued messages. It is especially troublesome during off-hours if patients must contend with a confusing recorded message.

- **Accessibility.** The logistics of office visits can be daunting, especially for elderly patients and parents with children. They may have difficulty parking. Once inside the building, particularly in a hospital, they may become easily confused by a multitude of elevator banks and look-alike hallways. If patients arrive for their appointment feeling disoriented from navigating the maze, this may add to their anxiety about a visit to the doctor.

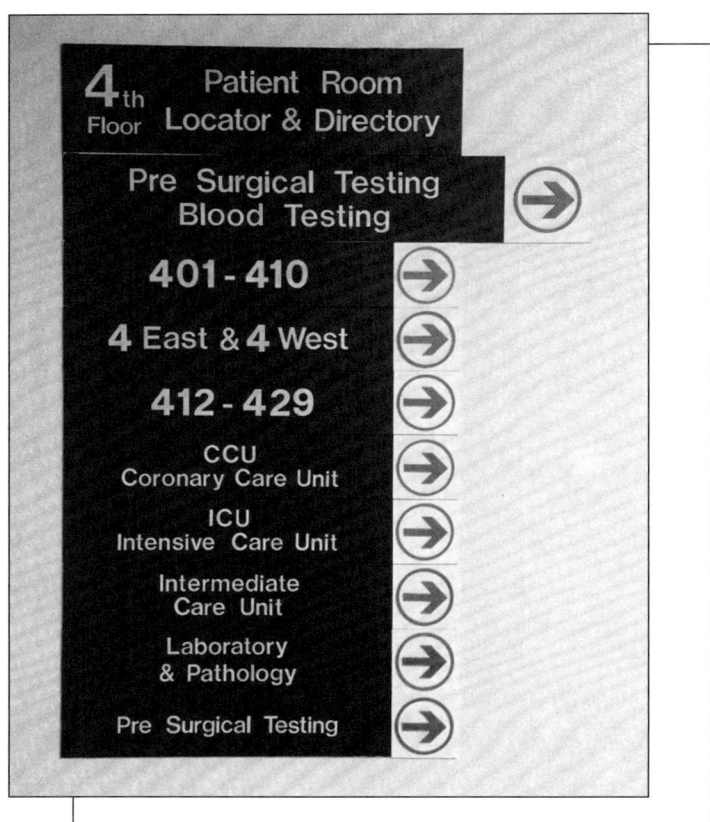

Physicians

Although the physician's role has been altered by managed care, it is still of primary importance in the delivery of quality health care. Even outside of the practice setting, hospitals depend on doctors for admissions; pharmaceutical companies seek their prescription endorsements; colleagues and allied health professionals look to them for referrals; and auxiliary health care facilities, such as nursing homes, home health care agencies, hospices, and rehabilitation centers, also rely on physician referrals. Patients increasingly look to their doctors for wellness information—to enable them to be active participants in both treatment and prevention of illness. So the physician's growing role as teacher can be especially satisfying.

Yet there is an inherent dichotomy in the day-to-day life of physicians. They can experience elation over their role in the healing process and distress over their limitations when a prognosis is terminal. They can experience the gratitude of patients, as well as their disappointments and anger.

Just who are these people who can contend with the paradoxical nature of medicine? Some characteristics they share in common are:

- They enjoy solving problems.
- They welcome interactions with people.
- They are emotionally committed to action.
- They try to balance their lives with humor.
- They display courage daily.

Gender Differences

According to an abstract, "*Calibrating the physician: personal awareness and effective patient care,*" in the August 13, 1997, issue of the *Journal of the American Medical Association*, there are specific differences between female and male physicians:

- Women MDs conduct longer patient visits, talk more, and use more communication strategies that are patient-centered and positive in approach; and
- They engage in preventive services more frequently and utilize a higher rate of screening for medical conditions.

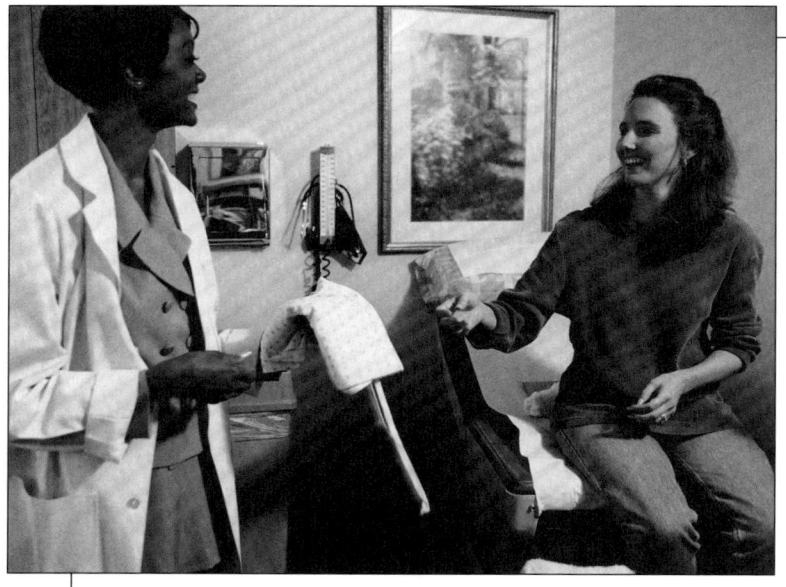

This is further corroborated in findings from the 1997 "Physician Worklife Study." A survey of 6,100 male and female physicians concludes that female physicians treat just as many complex medical problems as do their male counterparts; but women doctors carry a heavier burden when it comes to psychosocial issues and wellness care. The study also determines that:

- Time pressure is the single most important impediment to satisfaction for both male and female physicians regardless of their specialty.

- Both male and female physicians who practice in HMOs report the greatest time pressures. This was particularly true of primary care providers who say they need up to 42 percent more time for new patients and up to 25 percent more time for follow-up visits.

- Compared to male doctors, female doctors appear to need more resources, such as support staff, to help them handle health maintenance and psychosocial issues.

- Women doctors indicate they have less control over workplace issues, such as scheduling, colleague referrals, and hospitalization of patients.

- Women physicians report "burnout" at a rate of 1.5 times higher than that reported by their male counterparts.

- The need to manage complex medical and psychosocial issues under time constraints causes many general internists to report job dissatisfaction.

It's not enough for a physician to "know thyself." Patients also want to know about a doctor's qualifications and background. New patients may want this information *before* even making an appointment. Therefore, they may ask the receptionist such questions as:

- Where did the doctor attend medical school? Is he board certified?
- How many patients does the doctor see in one day (on average)?
- How far in advance must I schedule a routine visit?
- In case of emergency, how is the doctor reached?
- What are the doctor's hospital affiliations?
- What is the doctor's fee for first-time visits? For subsequent routine visits?

Such questions generally do not end with the receptionist. When patients come face-to-face with the doctor, there may be other queries ranging from: *"How do you keep up with the latest medical developments?"* to *"What is your view on second opinions?"* The doctors' responses, as well as their attitude and composure, help establish the rapport needed for a committed patient relationship.

The Importance of Ancillary Staff

There is no substitute for support staff that is accommodating, courteous and respectful of patients. These personnel—receptionists, physician assistants, nurses, lab technicians, billing clerks—can help prevent communication breakdowns with the patient.

Support staff must be prepared to resolve conflicts and handle complaints. In many practices, the office staff acts as intermediary between the patient and doctor, fielding questions, sometimes even providing answers. Staff also may be responsible for supplying education materials to patients and ensuring that they have, and understand, their home-care instructions.

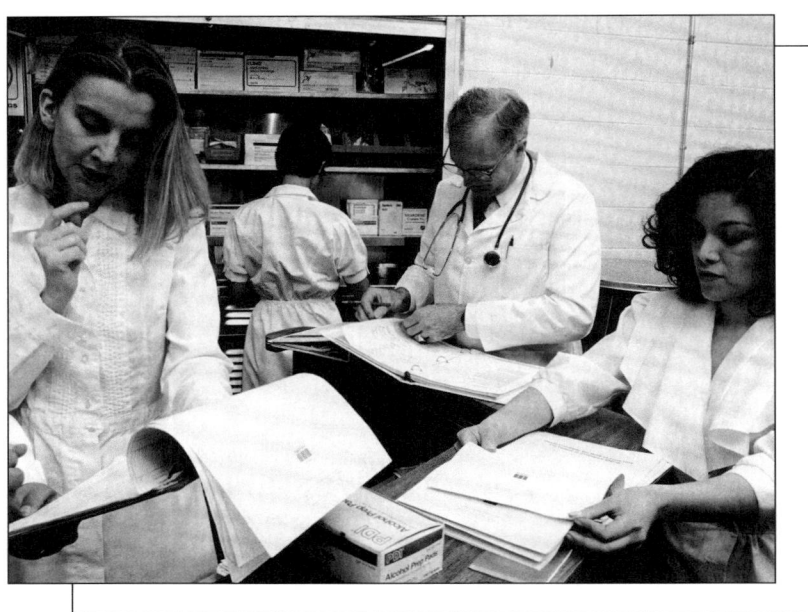

Physicians' Point of View

In response to the obstacles to good relations raised by patients, doctors might say:

"I, too, am overwhelmed by the amount of paperwork involved with patient visits."

"Some of my patients make last minute appointments, then complain about waiting."

"I give my patients information, but they don't follow up with it."

But these arguments are counterproductive. Instead, the focus should be on how to remove obstacles to good patient relations. In a May 1996 article in *American Medical News*, author Jane Oliva suggests the following:

- **Map out patient flow.** The patient experience in the office should be calm and undisrupted. Not only does an orderly flow of patients improve the work environment for physicians and staff, it is the key to patient satisfaction. Put systems and protocols in place to manage patient flow. For example, standardize exams as much as possible without hindering individualized care; conform exam room configurations; establish a uniform discharge procedure. Be consistent in these routines, so patients and staff know what to expect.

- *Reduce conflicting assignments.* Define and monitor the interactive time between physician and patient, and stress quality with that time to increase patient satisfaction. Eliminate all unnecessary interruptions such as unrelated paperwork and non-urgent phone calls.

- *Spend more time face to face.* Schedule realistically so that physicians and staff are not rushed, and then stick to it. Anticipate emergencies, and set up standard procedures for handling the unexpected. Extend on-call duty to office hours, not just nights and weekends, and make sure the on-call doctor has slots available to take people who must be seen immediately. Consider using nurse practitioners and physician assistants for routine screening. The challenge is to schedule for, and manage smoothly, two patient-flow tracks—routine health care and episodic care—so that one doesn't derail the other.

- *Streamline administrative function.* Set up a system for patients to call a separate number for refills, referrals, billing questions, and the like. Assign such tasks to staff who do not have to attend to patient-care responsibilities simultaneously.

- *Improve accessibility.* Make the effort to minimize excessive delays for the patient when scheduling appointments. Whenever possible, offer same-day appointments for special situations.

- *Respect the patient's time.* Do not leave the patient waiting interminably. Establish a maximum for time spent in the waiting room and, if the time spent threatens to surpass this limit, offer the patient an alternative slot or the option of seeing a different doctor, if possible. Set up parameters so that staff can act without physician approval. Encourage staff to troubleshoot with patients who might be angry or upset. Remember that in today's hectic world, your patient's time is precious, too.

- *Seek patient input.* Try suggestion boxes or comment forms; broach the subject of satisfaction with your patients, and then act on suggestions for change, whether it be delivery of health care, hours of operation, or staff support. If there are circumstances beyond your control, acknowledge the problem. For instance, if the issue is parking, have your staff forewarn patients so that they can allow for extra time.

Strengthening the integrity of the patient-physician relationship is key to the viability of your practice. The pointers contained in this chapter will help improve the relationship by encouraging patient trust and good will.

Laying the Groundwork

From the patient's perspective, doctors still have power over the relationship. Not only do they have more knowledge and more responsibility over outcome, but also it is they who set the ground rules. Small misunderstandings on either the physician or patient's part can lead to dissatisfaction; and these are more likely to occur when there are too many barriers to open, honest communication within the medical setting.

Just what are patients unhappy about?

An article, "*Consumer Complaint Department,*" which appeared in the April 1997 issue of the newsletter, *People's Medical Society,* reported that 125 of the 688 people surveyed voiced complaints about office visits to their doctor when expectations had not been met. Thirty percent of them were not happy with some aspect of the examination; 28 percent were concerned about the diagnostic tests ordered; 26 percent were not satisfied with the way their medical history was taken; 23 percent believed the doctor was not prepared for the visit; and 15 percent were displeased with the doctor/patient communication.

Other sources report that, by and large, patients' complaints focus on personal interactions with physicians rather than criticism of their clinical judgment, knowledge or experience. In the past, clinical ineptness would more likely drive a patient to seek a new doctor. Yet today they may seek a new doctor over the issue of interpersonal skills.

"Too many people settle for an unsatisfactory relationship with their doctor," suggests Warren M. Hoffman, in a text published in 1997 by the Society for Advancement of Education. Hoffman reported on a survey that showed most patients require a physician to demonstrate a combination of clinical and communication skills to prevent them from making a change. *The following eight factors are ranked according to their importance to patients:*

1. Does your doctor treat you as a whole person?

2. Does your doctor listen?

3. Does your doctor acknowledge your emotional needs?

4. Does your doctor look you in the eye?

5. Does your doctor explain treatment recommendations?

6. Does your doctor give you choices?

7. Does your doctor return your phone calls?

8. Does your doctor comfort you?

Resolving Bad Relationships. Medical treatment is an emotional experience not only for patients and their families, but for their physicians as well. Doctors must contend with their own reactions to patients' limitations, such as cognitive impairment, language barriers, socioeconomic factors, and physical disabilities.

In the March 31, 1998, issue of *The New York Times*, Abigail Zuger writes, "Doctors are now slowly beginning to submit their own professional interactions to the same kind of grueling analysis and repair work that other couples have undergone." She quotes Dr. William Sledge, a psychiatrist at the Yale University School of Medicine as saying, "They (doctors) should be aware of their reactions to patients, and realize that when a particular kind of patient repeatedly turns into a 'problem patient' for them, the doctor may be the one with the problem."

Physicians who can overcome difficult relationships are characterized as good problem solvers, satisfied in knowing they are helpful and able to avoid risk. They are tireless and selfless, strong believers that technology can cure human suffering. They further expect that patients will share these values.

It is important to remember that breakdowns in this relationship are not unilateral. When patients are not happy with doctors, the doctors are probably not happy with them.

Malpractice Prevention. A survey published in the February 19, 1997, issue of the *Journal of the American Medical Association* observed 59 primary physicians and 65 general surgeons. The survey showed that primary physicians who had no prior malpractice claims were more likely to tell patients what to expect during an office visit, spend more time with them, ask them more questions, and provide more encouragement. They also used humor whenever possible.

According to the authors of *Interviewing and Helping Skills for Health Care Professionals*, when barriers are placed in the patient-physician relationship—such as technical advances, geographic distances or lack of interpersonal skills—malpractice action becomes more likely. When such barriers do exist in a practice setting, the book offers these tips to help prevent malpractice suits:

- *Communication and interpersonal skills.* When physicians build emotional ties with patients, through communication and interaction, they may have the key to malpractice prevention. *Patients show reluctance to sue a doctor with whom they have a good rapport.*

- *Accessibility.* A long wait in the doctor's office without explanation or apology from staff, failure to return calls or delays in returning them, rushed examinations with no time for questions—these all show a lack of concern about the patient. *Common courtesy can be the answer to patient satisfaction.*

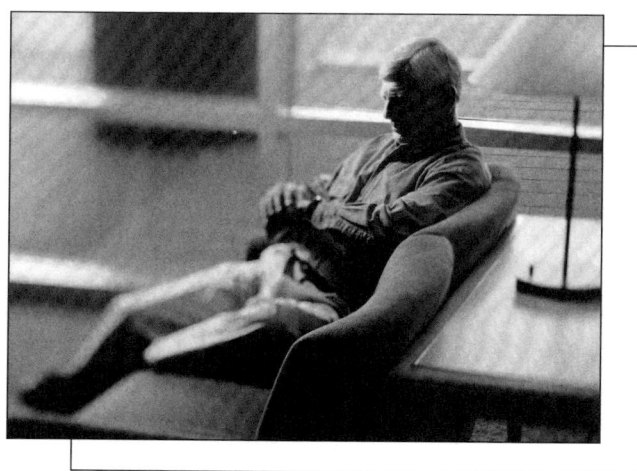

- *Fees.* When fees appear unjustifiably high, lawsuits may prevail. *Initiating discussion about fees and/or arrangements for monthly payments may make the difference.*

- *Ancillary staff.* When staff deals with patients, a lack of courtesy, sensitivity, and regard for privacy can result in liability. *There is no substitute for pleasant personnel who go out of their way to make patients feel that their problems and concerns are important.*

- *Due care.* Suggesting treatment protocols that are not generally accepted, not following up on patients' progress when they've been referred to specialists, and failing to seek other options when a regimen is not working can be viewed as an invitation to file a professional negligence action. Furthermore, writing a prescription that leads to medical complications opens the physician to potential liability. *Attention to details, caution, and follow up are more likely to lead to favorable outcomes.*

- **Patient rights.** Medical procedures should be explained and those that are experimental should be identified. Patients should be informed of any attendant discomfort, risks, or benefits involved, appropriate alternative procedures, and all of their related questions should be answered. They also should have knowledge of their right to withdraw or discontinue treatment. *If patients are informed and able to participate in making decisions about their care, they are unlikely to bring lawsuits.*

More Steps to Improved Physician-Patient Relations

Unfortunately, the patient-physician relationship is not taught in medical schools and residency programs. In years past, physicians have had to learn from experience what their relationship with patients should be. As a new generation of patients expects good relations at the outset, having the skills to establish good will are more important than ever. The following tactics will help in this regard:

Personal awareness. A lack of personal awareness in physicians regarding their own life experiences, values, beliefs, attitudes, and biases can hamper how they interact with patients. What used to be called "bedside manner" can have a profound effect on patients. If that "manner" is less than gracious, it can lead to professional censure or even malpractice suits. Shortcomings in personal awareness also can lead to burnout for physicians. Fortunately, there are appropriate settings for addressing these issues, whether in a psychiatrist's office, support group, one-on-one with colleagues, or stress-reducing sessions at the gym. Any positive coping mechanism can help physicians build satisfaction both in themselves and their patients.

Empathy. Empathy may serve as the bridge between physician and patient. It refers to the ability of physicians to put themselves "in the shoes" of their patients. Why empathy? In the January 1996 issue of the *Archives of Internal Medicine*, author Dean Gianakos says, "First, empathy allows the physician to gain additional knowledge or insight about the patient." With this newfound knowledge, physicians can become more in tune with patients' emotional needs and therefore help them make decisions about their health care. "Second," Gianakos continues, "empathy may engender feelings of affection and tenderness toward the patient, feelings that prompt caring and tender actions that in turn foster healing." At the very least, patients may have some relief for their emotional suffering. He sums up by saying that the understanding physicians acquire through empathy is like a "moral compass." Empathy helps them treat patients as they (physicians) would like to be treated in the same circumstances.

Negotiation. Often the problems and issues in a difficult patient-physician relationship can be negotiated. An article on effective relationships in the July 7, 1997, *American Medical News*, authored by Leonard J. Marcus and Barry C. Dorn, highlights the importance of "viewing the patient-physician interaction as a negotiation, especially during a time of managed care and capitated reimbursement." The authors go on to list several characteristics of the physician in negotiation with a patient:

- Be an active listener—"I understand what you mean."
- Experience their pain and/or concern.
- Obtain patients' "buy-in" to their treatment plan by giving them the information they need to participate on equal terms.

Negotiation doesn't stop with patient visits. Today's physicians must be prepared to negotiate on behalf of patients with managed care plans, other health care professionals providing consultation or services, hospital administration, and clinical hospital staff.

Test Yourself

How many of these characteristics describe your practice?

As a physician:

- ☐ I treat human beings, not patients.
- ☐ I act competently and am consistent, dependable, and trustworthy when dealing with my patients.
- ☐ I communicate clearly and make sure my patients understand everything I have said.
- ☐ I practice active listening and acknowledge my patients' worries and concerns.
- ☐ I maintain a positive attitude toward my patients.
- ☐ I try to empathize with my patient's experience of their condition, and then I communicate my understanding.
- ☐ I give appropriate and useful information, advise patients of their options, and help them select the best alternative.
- ☐ I am aware of my own needs and keep them separate from those of my patients.

In dealing with patients, my staff:

- ☐ Is friendly, understanding and concerned.
- ☐ Treats them with courtesy and politeness.
- ☐ Respects their privacy and confidentiality.
- ☐ Explains office procedures.
- ☐ Communicates any delays.
- ☐ Offers information and facilitates the filling of prescriptions.
- ☐ Encourages them to call if they have any questions.

Section 2

Increasing Patient Satisfaction

Offering Solutions

There have been thousands of published studies to define patient satisfaction and determine its impact on physicians. When patients are satisfied with the services of their doctors, long-term relationships are almost always assured. When they communicate that satisfaction to family and friends, new patients may result.

Because patients' ratings of satisfaction are naturally subjective, there has been a divergence in the approach to the studies. In some studies, patient characteristics such as needs and attitudes are held most relevant; in other studies, sociodemographic characteristics are considered the key.

A patient satisfaction study reported in an article in the Winter 1995 edition of the *Journal of Healthcare Marketing* used patient sociodemographics and linked them to patients' perceptions of the quality of care they have received. Applying characteristics such as sex, age, occupation, education and income, the study showed that only age and education had a significant effect. The researchers concluded that to improve patient satisfaction, less emphasis should be placed on patient's sociodemographic characteristics and more placed on delivery of services.

This is directly opposite the approach taken by the health care marketing professionals of the 1980s and 90s, who emphasized the demographic differences of the "new health care consumer." They suggested segmenting this consumer market and assessing each segment so that hospitals and doctors know what their patients really want.

Whatever their point-of-view, health-care marketing and research mavens do agree that age, education and demographic changes—such as households with both parents working and the growing number of single parents—have notable impact on patient satisfaction.

According to the book, *Communicating with Medical Patients*, edited by Moira Stewart and Debra Roter, there are many aspects of the physician-patient relationship that lead to patient satisfaction. They report that an important relationship exists between patient satisfaction and physician warmth, sensitivity, and eye contact. Other factors relate to direct communication between doctors and patients—sharing opinions, answering questions, and exchanging information.

For the purposes of this book, indicators of patient satisfaction are categorized under three headings: *Convenience and Service*; *Autonomy and Control*; *Interaction and Communication.*

Convenience and Service

In her book, *Market-Driven Health Care*, Regina E. Herzlinger writes that convenience has substantially raised the number of patient visits to a doctor. "For example," she says, "a provider who is available on weekends or evenings . . . increased the number of visits by 16 percent." What the physician charges is less of a variable than convenience, Herzlinger states.

What do patients think when they are asked to rate the service provided in the hospital or doctor's office? Courtesy from a nurse or help from the receptionist in filing insurance claims may elicit a positive response. In relation to doctors, availability or bedside manner might be the determining factor.

A table that appears in the book, *The Healthcare Customer Service Revolution*, by David and Peggy Zimmerman and Charles Lund, shows how patients define the importance of service in relation to their physicians.

What Patient Wants	National Average	Older Patients (over 55)	Middle-aged Patients (36-55)	Younger Patients (under 35)
Shorter wait time	52.3%	60 %	43.3%	46.7%
Friendliness of staff	41.9	42.5	33.3	60.0
Communication	44.2	37.5	56.7	40.0
Compassion	38.4	35.0	43.3	46.7
Professionalism	19.8	17.5	16.7	33.4
Efficiency	10.5	15.0	6.7	6.7
Accuracy	7.0	12.5	3.3	6.7
Privacy	3.5	5.0	3.3	3.1

It's not news to health care researchers that most patients are not always able to assess the quality of care they have received, but they are able to rate the amenities provided in the hospital and in doctors' offices. Some other aspects of convenience and service that patients might rate as priorities are:

- **Reasonable location.** Patients seek out doctors located fairly close to where they reside or near public transit. Those that drive expect convenient parking. Whatever the mode of transportation, the receptionist should provide clear directions when the appointment is set.

- **Flexible scheduling.** Appointment schedules that cut some daytime hours and add evening and/or Saturday hours meet patients' needs without imposing additionally on doctors, many of whom already work long days. Since most patients want an appointment as quickly as possible, especially when they are anxious about their symptoms, the receptionist should ask whether a particular day of the week, time of day or the next available appointment is the priority. If the doctor is significantly behind schedule, it is important that staff try to notify patients beforehand. If the patient has already arrived, then an explanation and apology for the delay should be provided.

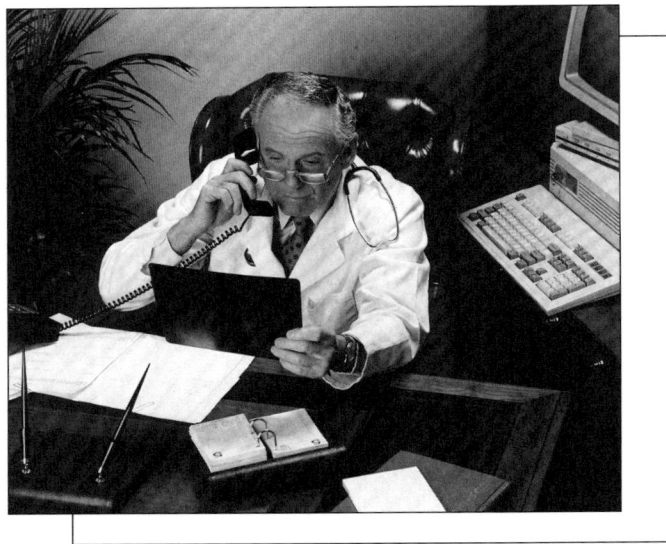

- **Prompt return of phone calls.** Most physicians have 24-hour telephone coverage. While the procedures for emergency and non-emergency calls vary from practice to practice, they should be communicated clearly to patients so they know exactly what to expect.

- **Emergency instructions.** Every opportunity should be taken to educate patients as to what constitutes an emergency and what procedures should be followed. Try to notify patients, particularly those undergoing treatment, when their doctor won't be available during regular office hours. Whenever possible, introduce your patients to covering physicians so they will not feel they are dealing with complete strangers.

- **Prescription policy.** Renewal or prescription of medications without an office visit will depend on state laws and the individual doctor's policy. Whatever that policy, communicate it clearly to patients.

Autonomy and Control

Both researchers and marketers agree that patients today are better educated and that this leads to self-determination and a desire for control when it comes to their health.

During the past 30 years, the percentage of people graduating from high school has risen from 50 to 80 percent. Mature adults are going back to school to receive a high school degree or to start or finish college. This acquisition of knowledge has made the population more confident about their decision-making abilities. No longer relying on experts, they are willing and able to research things for themselves.

Health-related topics are broadcast frequently on the radio and TV, and newspapers and magazines regularly report the latest developments. With the advent of computers and online search programs, patients easily access "authoritative" information. Yet in the June 11th edition of the *Chicago Tribune* an Ohio University study reported that, despite its vast resources of medical information, the Internet may contain much that is unreliable ("Beware of online info"). Researchers analyzed 30 computer articles on a childhood illness and found that only 20 percent of them offered correct information. Some of the information was even deemed potentially harmful.

In today's media-saturated environment, doctors and patients need to form an alliance that combines the physician's expertise, technical knowledge and skill with the need of the patient to participate in all matters concerning personal health. Every interaction between doctor and patient requires an exchange of information, hope, confidence, and credibility.

Doctors may take a more proactive position by offering patients:

- A clear explanation of diagnosis, medications and prognosis.
- Respect for their opinions about their health problems.
- Acknowledgment of their concerns.
- Reports on normal as well as abnormal test results.
- Full and open answers to questions.
- Discussion of differing treatment options.
- Direction for seeking expert advice and second opinions.
- A willingness to concur on decisions and treatment.
- Coordination with other service providers.

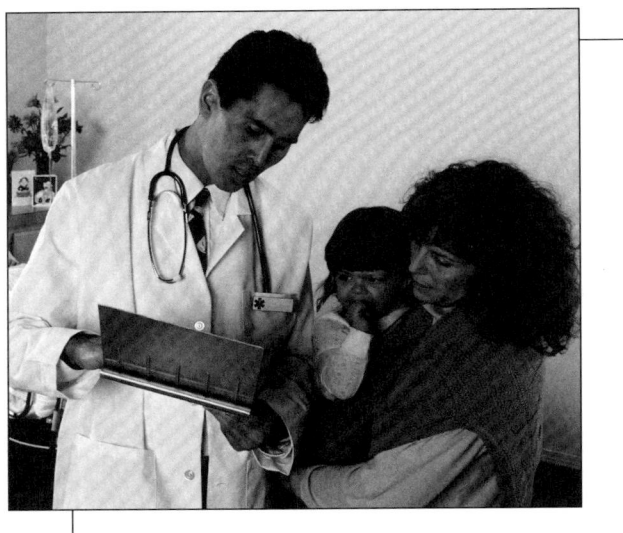

Interaction and Communication

Interaction and communication set the stage for long-lasting relationships between doctors and patients and are vital elements of patient satisfaction and retention. Without this give and take, the curtain closes before the play begins.

Patients unanimously want to feel that doctors are truly interested in them. They want their undivided attention. They want compassion. Translated into action, patients commonly expect a physician to:

- Acknowledge them prior to the examination, referring to them by name.
- Demonstrate a knowledge of their personal and family history.
- Display a sense of humor.
- Inquire about a range of their concerns.
- Listen to what they say intently.
- Apologize and explain any interruptions.
- Visibly wash hands before contact.
- Carefully and gently conduct the examination.

A survey of 1500 patients and doctors, conducted by the Bayer Institute for Health Care Communication, suggests that patients who rated communications with their physicians as excellent were four times more likely to believe they had received excellent health care than those who did not. In many ways, communication may be more important to the physician-patient relationship than a doctor's skill. It can have more influence on the patient outcomes—health and satisfaction—and on the doctor's reputation.

Further evidence of the importance of communication comes from a Johns Hopkins University study published in the *Journal of the American Medical Association*, (Jan. 22/29, 1997.) The study looked at the different communication styles of physicians and polled both doctors and patients about their preferences. The researchers analyzed the conversations between 127 physicians and 527 patients.

They found:

- In 32 percent of the visits, doctors asked simple yes-and-no questions and primarily used medical jargon to communicate.
- In 33 percent of the visits, this communication style was combined with slightly more personal conversation.
- Twenty percent of visits involved equal amounts of medical talk and personal conversation.
- Eight percent of the conversations were dominated by personal exchanges—small talk, encouraging phrases, and open-ended questions about lifestyle and general well-being.
- Another eight percent of conversations were categorized as "consumerist." In this style, patients were expected to ask questions and the physician to provide all available information.

Patients were most satisfied when doctors asked the questions and did most of the talking. Physicians preferred the "consumerist" style, with patients doing most of the talking.

Tips on Building Communication Skills

Concentrate on the positive. For instance, (if they complain about the long wait) tell patients you appreciate their patience, then move quickly to the next subject.

Sit down. Patients will have the perception you are spending more time with them than if you stand during the visit.

Try not to hurry the patient. Interrupt only if their explanation of their health concern is too lengthy.

Encourage patients to make lists. It puts them more at ease and helps them cite efficiently questions they want to ask.

Listen carefully. Repeat what patients have said so they know you have understood.

Ask for clarification. Precise information will make your job that much simpler.

Don't wait for the patient to bring up every concern. It's not uncommon for patients to think of more problems and questions after they have left the office.

Display confidence. Outline a plan and tell patients what they can expect.

Offer choices whenever possible. Let patients take part in decision-making, particularly when there are treatment alternatives.

Encourage further contact. Tell patients you or your nurse will be available to answer additional questions if the need arises.

Communicating Bad News

At no time is communication more important than when telling patients they have a life-threatening disease, deteriorating condition or terminal illness. Because physicians are not always trained for these circumstances, they may be as unprepared as their patients. Also, many physicians view death as a personal or professional failure.

At this time of bad news, all of the physician's interactive skills are brought to bear. Patients require the physician's time, attention, expertise and on-going concern. While the majority of patients want to be free of pain and want to die at home, studies have shown their wishes are often not heeded.

In an article published in *The New York Times* (December 23, 1997), entitled "Forget About Bedside Manners, Some Doctors Have No Manners," Susan Gilbert writes that doctors still have a hard time breaking bad news, particularly when the patient is a child. This fact is attributed to a lack of training in medical school, although there is more training in communication today than there was a decade ago. The article refers to guidelines published in medical literature on the subject of discussing bad news with patients. These guidelines include conveying the information clearly and privately, without interruptions from colleagues or beepers, and in most cases, with members of the family present.

Families are important. In this same article, Dr. C. Everett Koop, former Surgeon General of the United States, is quoted as saying, "Nobody in medicine enjoys talking to the families about problems that include death. On the other hand, the physician who is able to give comfort to a family accomplishes so much. The only way for a doctor to master this is to do it over and over again."

Medical History

Often the first communication patients have with their doctors is when they are asked their medical history. The extent to which medical history is useful depends on the kinds of questions included on the written form, usually completed by the patient in the waiting room, and during the face-to-face interview with the doctor in the examination room. When the medical history is really effective, it will give insight into the patient's personal life, attitude and psychological state. Most importantly, it will help the doctor in future relations with the patient, including making accurate diagnoses.

In addition to the standard medical history questions, the following queries can give the physician valuable information about the patient:

- Do you feel nervous about coming to the doctor? If so, what is your biggest concern?
- When was your last physical examination? Do you see a doctor regularly for checkups or go on an as-needed basis?
- Do you drink or smoke? If so, how would you describe your habit?
- What is your occupation? Are you currently under stress at work?
- Is your home life fairly stable? Any specific worries?
- Do you have children? How old are they, and how are they doing?
- Is your sex life satisfactory?
- In what ways would you like to better your health?

- Are you handling any harmful chemicals on the job or at home?
- Do you take any nutritional supplements?
- What do you do to relax?

Other Ways to Stay in Touch with Patients

- **Tickler files** that indicate when patients are due for checkups and generate postcards as reminders of this and any other timely information
- **Flyers** to ensure that all patients are made aware of what services are offered
- **Brochures** that contain a short resume and photo of the physician members of a group practice or clinic
- **Newsletters** that highlight prevention information and announce new services and additions or changes to the office staff
- **Patient education materials** that explain an illness, list its symptoms, discuss treatment, and describe medications and their side effects
- **Printed instruction sheets** that may be personalized to meet individual patient needs
- **Suggestion boxes** placed strategically in the waiting room

Communications to Generate New Patients

In today's health care environment, it has become acceptable for doctors to market themselves. To an extent, they did this in the past through referrals from colleagues. Now physicians can list themselves on referral services offered to the public by hospitals and fee-for-service organizations. These services are a convenience for patients seeking a doctor, as well as a marketing tool for doctors to communicate their qualifications and availability.

For many people, physicians included, marketing is advertising, and the cost of advertising can be prohibitive. However, many physicians are taking advantage of less expensive marketing tools:

Newspaper ads. Newspapers are accessible, affordable, and credible. In most metropolitan areas, daily newspapers have local editions. Other weekly and monthly papers are geared to target populations based on age, gender, business or recreational interest. Local newspapers published in suburban areas or in small towns have the added advantage of being right in the doctor's backyard.

Public relations. Doctors can gain visibility in the public eye by serving on charitable committees, donating their time to local civic groups, serving as an authority for medical news, and working on government research projects.

Community outreach. Each year, thousands of prospective patients attend health-related events such as seminars and health fairs sponsored by local hospitals, libraries and other civic groups. Though time-consuming, taking part in these events can be most effective for doctors.

Communicating by Computer

Doctors have relied on computers for billing purposes for years, but it's only in recent times that computers have been utilized to keep track of patient health. A small group of physicians affiliated with Northwestern University, Chicago, have been demonstrating the benefits of computerized patient records. Besides making information easier to access, computers can be programmed to notify patients who are likely to forget about flu shots or various other annual or biannual tests. Because records can be accessed from the office or home, covering physicians are privy to more hands-on information when an emergency arises. Once doctors become adept at updating patient records on the computer, they find it easier to formulate extensive health histories, enter new symptoms, renew prescriptions, and implement patient education. For doctors with notoriously bad handwriting, computers are a decided advantage.

Malpractice and Communication

Reports increasingly indicate that malpractice suits are typically triggered by a failure to communicate rather than a negligent act itself. The complaints of those who are generally happy with the patient-physician relationship are usually easily resolved with a minimum of effort or change.

The Society for the Advancement of Education reported in the October 1997 issue of *USA Today* that the primary reason patients with bad outcomes sue for malpractice is not lapse in quality of care or medical negligence, but how physicians talk with patients. Process and tone was found to be even more important than what they say. Simple things like listening to patients and showing concern, orienting patients to what they can expect during a visit, or checking to see that patients understand instructions can make a difference.

Assessing Patient Satisfaction

Patient assessment tools offer an excellent opportunity for providers to determine what satisfies patients—what they really want. If a survey is properly structured, doctors can retrieve information that helps them improve their current services and determine new services to meet patient needs.

In "How to get the best reading of patient satisfaction," an article in the July 15, 1996 issue of *Medical Economics*, Ken Terry writes, "Group practices are measuring patient satisfaction as never before. Competition and pressure from health plan and employers are the two main reasons. Also, employers are demanding data on 'quality'—and patient satisfaction is the most accessible quality measure."

Terry outlines the issues in designing and conducting patient satisfaction surveys, based on advice from experts in the field:

Who Should Design the Survey? Some groups with less than 50 physicians try to design the surveys themselves. Frequently these surveys are merely left for patients to find in the waiting room. At most they contain a few check-off items and very little room for comments. Medium- and large-size practices that use surveys today employ research companies or consultants, many of which have the added benefit of national databases for comparison of patient satisfaction in practices of similar size.

Depending on what information the practice is seeking, these research professionals develop surveys containing questions on specific areas of concern. The American College of Physicians/American Society of Internal Medicine has designed a survey of 81 questions. Unlike other surveys, it focuses on the physician, because the College feels that including other office staff doesn't tell doctors enough about their own performance in relation to patient satisfaction.

Is There a Best Way to Survey? There are a variety of methods used to conduct surveys, including:

Mail. Results of return by mail surveys vary from 20 to 40 percent. Sometimes an incentive is enclosed (as little as 25 cents and up to a dollar). Reminder postcards that follow up the survey mailing also are effective. The major benefit of a mail survey is that it allows patients to remain anonymous if they choose, and it gives them time at home to reflect on the quality of their visit. However, with the cost of postage, mail surveys can be expensive, especially if returns are low.

Telephone. Some companies doubt that telephone polls give reliable data because of "interview bias." The interviewer's approach or a patient's annoyance when interrupted by a phone call, especially at dinnertime or late in the evening, may affect the answers. Phone surveys also can be costly, especially when physician-specific data is the focus. Studies show that patients generally rate doctors higher in telephone surveys as opposed to other surveying methods.

In-office. This type of survey (the most cost effective of research methods) asks as little as two questions per key area. The patient circles a rating (for example, 1 to 4; 1 being poor, 2, fair, 3, good, 4, excellent) as to practice performance. Expecting all patients to remain in the office after a visit to fill out a survey may be asking too much. Some practices randomly select patients and ask them to begin working on the survey while in the waiting room prior to their visit. Although patients do not have to include their names on in-office surveys, they may feel a lack of privacy when they are filling them out under scrutiny of office staff. They also may be less able to express their true feelings right after their visit with the doctor.

Focus groups. Because it is prohibitively expensive to reach a wide number of patients in focus groups, this method is used primarily to ascertain and fine-tune what questions to ask when doing mail, telephone or in-office surveys.

Groups may achieve better results by using a combination of survey tactics. For instance, in-office surveys for current patients may be used in conjunction with surveys mailed to patients who haven't been in the office for some time. Whatever methods are used, patients should be made aware that the survey comes from their doctor's office and has their doctor's approval. In all cases, doctors should be kept up-to-date on survey development and implementation.

One caveat, however, is that a badly constructed and administered survey can result in data that ranges from slightly off the mark to completely wrong. If you are not familiar with survey technique, check with your state medical society, the marketing department at your local hospital (which may be delighted to help you survey patients, especially if you're willing to share the data), or the marketing arm of a managed care organization with which you have a contract.

How Large a Survey Sample is Needed? Statistically there should be at least 50-75 responses per doctor in a 12-month period to make surveying meaningful. This doesn't necessarily apply to a single survey—it could be the result of multiple surveys conducted in a designated time frame.

The other factor in choosing the number of patients to sample is the expected response rate. Telephone polls usually get a response of 50 percent or better; mail, as previously mentioned, gets about 20 to 40 percent; and in-house rates vary greatly.

How Often Should Surveys be Conducted? Continuous surveys may be needed to gather enough meaningful data on patient satisfaction to review performance or improve quality. However, there are some groups that choose to act immediately on data they collect from recent patients.

To decide how often to conduct surveys, a group's objectives for doing a survey should be clearly stated up front, and there should be funds available to reach those goals.

How Much Will the Survey Cost? According to Jerry Seibert of the Chicago-based Parkside Associates, a quarterly mail survey for a 12-doctor group could cost $5,000 to $15,000 annually, assuming 1200 patients were canvassed per quarter and there was a 50 percent response. That breaks down to $2 to $6 per response. A telephone survey would cost somewhere between $11 and $15 per response.

What Kinds of Issues and Concerns Should a Survey Cover? A sample survey might include:

- Overall quality of care
- Ease in making appointments
- Waiting time in office
- Convenience of location
- Convenience of hours

- Availability of public transportation
- Atmosphere of office
- Respect of patient's privacy
- Attitude of receptionist
- In-house lab facilities and equipment
- Professionalism of technicians
- Helpfulness and friendliness of nurse
- Time spent with physician
- Thoroughness of examination
- Doctor's courtesy and consideration
- Treatment options presented
- Encouragement of preventive care
- Clear instructions for medication and treatment
- Telephone access to doctor

Dissatisfied patients are often demanding and critical. They tend to make each encounter a negative one for their caregivers and themselves. On the other hand, patients who are highly satisfied are more likely to comply with physician advice, take an active role in their care, and achieve better outcomes.

Conducting surveys might seem like a great deal of work and expense. But if the results bring about changes that improve quality, the use of surveys can enhance patient satisfaction. Assessment tools can help doctors and patients alike.

Section 3

Assuring Patient Retention and Loyalty

The Role of Choice

With managed care, patients' ability to choose their health care plans and their doctors has become increasingly limited. Senior citizens still have options in selecting a Medicare supplementary insurance plan; thus, they have some leeway in making a switch. However, employees covered in the workplace have fewer choices. When they aren't happy with their health care, their only alternative is to complain to their employers.

In the February 24, 1997, issue of *American Medical News*, Susan Keane Baker suggests some service-oriented practices to help limit complaints and improve patient retention rates:

- ***Staff knows patients and their health situation.*** Staff can review the daily appointment list so they recognize patients by name and have some knowledge about the reason for their visit. It discourages patients if their name is continually mispronounced or they are asked the purpose of their visit, particularly if other patients can overhear.

- ***Staff makes things easier for the patient.*** Physicians should establish a "patients first" policy and hire staff with the people skills to put it into action. Patients will recognize and appreciate staff efforts if they go out of their way for them.

- ***Physicians and staff explain what is going to happen and why.*** It's important to relate the "whys and wherefores" so patients know in advance what procedures will be performed. For instance, if a patient comes in for an injured hand, the nurse should explain beforehand that the doctor will first check his vital signs. Simply asking this patient to "strip to the waist" will in no way put him at ease.

- **Systems are improved for patient convenience.** Systems can be a concern for patients and staff alike. Staff members should be encouraged to suggest changes if systems prevent them from serving patients efficiently and humanely. Likewise, patients should be surveyed regularly. When systems that create confusion and frustration are identified, they should be corrected.

- **Patients are not kept waiting.** Long waits in the doctor's office have been recognized as one of patients' primary grievances. Amenities such as telephones, light snacks, good reading materials, and comfortable surroundings can help. Most important, staff should communicate to the patient the length and reason for the wait, offer to reschedule an appointment, or designate a time to return later in the day, which recognizes the patients "place" in the schedule. These actions will demonstrate respect for the patient's time.

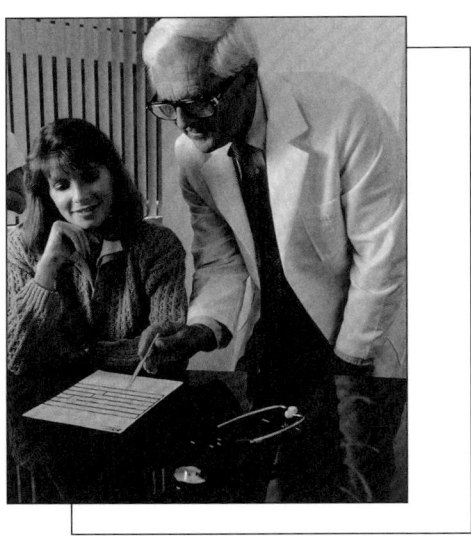

- **Forms are readable.** Readability of forms depends not only on printing quality, but also on how well questions have been constructed. A simple "yes" or "no" question may be confusing when a range of answers might apply. Many forms also require information patients may not have on hand. Both new and existing patients should be reminded ahead of time to bring any information relevant to this paperwork.

- *Important information is in writing.* There are two kinds of information patients may need. One is immediate—including prescriptions, directions for care, date of next visit, etc. The other might be general information about an illness or preventive health care. To avoid questions at a later date, doctors or staff members should write down immediate information as clearly and concisely as possible and review it with patients to make sure it is understood. Patients who require general information should be given a written list of available resources.

- *The privacy of patients is upheld.* Violation of privacy ranks high among patient complaints. Procedures to preserve privacy include: knocking on the door before entering the examination room; having garments and/or sheets available for cover up; getting permission from patients for having more than one doctor and nurse present during an exam; requiring patients to remove clothing only once during the visit; and allowing patients to dress before meeting with the doctor when the examination is finished.

- *Billing procedures and billing statements can be easily understood.* Staff should be prepared to clearly answer patient inquiries regarding charges for visits and tests. Prior to the first visit, new patients should be given complete information about billing requirements and the accepted method of payment. Actual billing statements should simply list each item of service and its cost, any outstanding charges, and then total due.

- *Voice mail is user friendly.* Many offices employ a voice mail system during office hours when phone lines are busy. Asking the caller to "please hold" or "leave a name and number" is fine if time on hold is limited and calls are returned in a timely fashion. The touch-tone technology of "branching" requires the caller to listen to a series of options and press the appropriate number according to the nature of the call. Simplifying instructions and limiting the number of options is the key to success with this type of system.

Understanding Patient Retention

According to Dawn Bendall and Thomas L. Powers, in the Winter 1995 edition of the *Journal of Health Care Marketing,* patient retention can be defined as the system by which health care providers influence patient satisfaction and loyalty and, therefore, maintain existing patients. Patient satisfaction is described as an attitude that arises from meeting or not meeting perceptions and expectations of quality care. When patient satisfaction is referred to as loyalty, it means that the intention of the patient after treatment is to return to the same health care provider.

The article goes on to report on a proposed patient retention model developed by the American Marketing Association. Although this model is particularly relevant to hospitals and managed care programs, it is also applies to physician group practices and networks that are looking for information on retention. Patient retention terms examined in the model include:

Patient Expectation Level. The expectations of patients can be criteria for which health care services are evaluated.

Whether or not services fall short, meet or exceed expectations, may likely determine patients' attitudes.

Patient Satisfaction Attitudes. These attitudes are formed from initial and subsequent reactions to the health care service that the patient receives. Whether the experience leaves the patient satisfied or dissatisfied will probably lead to word-of-mouth communications about the provider that are either positive (recommendation) or negative (complaint).

Time Lag. Patients' initial reactions to a health service they have received may be affected over time. If there is positive communication from the provider during the time lag, attitudes may be influenced for the better.

Quality Perception. Patients who perceive that a high quality of care was delivered are likely to return to the provider for future care.

Provider Communications. There is little doubt that patients' attitudes can be affected by provider communications, particularly if they occur during the time of service or shortly thereafter. It may be as simple as expressing concern for the patient during the visit or providing follow-up information, such as test results, within the promised time.

Word-of-Mouth Referrals. Patients who develop positive feelings about a health care encounter will most likely return and recommend that provider to others.

Complaint Resolution. If patients form a negative attitude about health care encounters, the handling of their complaints will influence their behavior. With sufficient resolution of the complaint, patients are more likely to change their negative attitudes and use the provider again.

Switching Doctors. The end result of patient dissatisfaction that cannot be resolved is that patients will seek a change to a new provider when future care is needed.

Patient Loyalty. Both initial and subsequent satisfaction attitudes are important factors in generating patient loyalty. Measuring patient satisfaction with in-office questionnaires may provide some early insight. If initial attitudes do not reflect satisfaction, efforts should be made to answer and resolve patients' complaints before too much time passes.

Patient Retention. The ultimate goal of any patient retention program is to generate positive attitudes that affect a patient's future behavior. The patient who intends to return most likely will recommend the provider to others.

In conclusion, the article states that more research is needed to understand the satisfaction and loyalty factors involved in patient retention. Successful research depends on health care providers trying harder to elicit patient dissatisfaction. When patients' negative feelings are comprehended, the opportunity for resolution arises. It is up to providers to take advantage of this critical chance to convert unhappy patients into loyal ones.

The Elusive Patient Loyalty

In his book, *Beyond Patient Satisfaction*, and in an article written for the Winter 1994 edition of the *Journal of Health Care Marketing*, R. Scott MacStravic states that the difficulty in defining patient loyalty is that there is no consensus on what the concept means. Over the years, authors knowledgeable on the subject have offered various definitions of patient loyalty. These authors describe patient loyalty as:

- An attitude.
- A commitment to the provider.
- Resistance to changing to another provider.
- Satisfaction with a practice rather than a specific encounter.
- Willingness to promote the provider's virtue.
- Intention to return to the same provider.
- Intention to recommend the provider to others.
- A pattern of behavior.

MacStravic reports that patient loyalty will save physicians the costs of trying to attract new patients and will lower health care costs because loyal patients listen to their doctors. He finds that care encounters with loyal patients have more satisfaction for physicians because these patients are likely to:

- Make timely appointments.
- Follow their advice.
- Take active roles in the treatment and prevention process.
- Have realistic expectations.
- Share more relevant information about their health.
- Use more preventive services.
- Communicate better outcomes.
- Report fewer complaints.
- Provide suggestions for existing or new services.
- Pay their bills.
- Help in finding new patients.

Possibly the most valuable contribution loyal patients can make to their doctors is in the area of public relations. Sharing some medical experience with relatives and friends or talking with other patients in the waiting room can give rise to new or stronger loyalties.

Finally, loyal patients are less likely to bring suits for malpractice against their doctors.

At the same time, their care creates greater profitability for doctors because loyal patients are easier to serve more efficiently.

For patients, loyalty to their doctor means:

- Enhanced quality through continuity of care.
- Savings on the cost of finding a new physician.
- Feelings of confidence and trust in their physician.
- Reduced anxiety when medical care is needed.
- Taking leadership roles in physician-organized patient support groups.

What Makes Patients Loyal?

According to MacStravic, measuring loyalty depends on what definition is used. Thus, there are widely differing opinions on how patient loyalty should be studied. Some experts feel that consistent use, actual recommendations of a physician, and provision of useful information in an exchange between patient and doctor are better indicators of loyalty and easier to evaluate than expressions of willingness or intentions.

National surveys have gathered a variety of statistics concerning who loyal patients are. Measured in terms of a usual or consistent source of medical care, one survey found 73 percent of respondents were loyal to a physician, HMO, clinic or other health care provider. Studies also show that women and older people, as well as married couples and people with chronic illnesses, are more loyal than men or younger people.

Other correlates of patient loyalty are:

- People who choose their own physician and use that physician's services over a period of time.
- People who perceive that their doctors are accessible, take enough time with them, express interest in their concerns, and receive complete and clear communications from them.
- People who feel full confidence in their doctors; and the doctors, in turn, treat them with respect.
- People who feel they have some control and an ability to make choices.
- People who make a commitment to the physician, such as providing a recommendation to potential patients.
- People who will tolerate inconvenience to continue to see that physician.

As perceived by patients, these are some of the positive attributes of physicians and their staff that generate loyalty:

- High quality of competence and skill.
- Genuine interest in their patients.
- Honest, reputable and trustworthy.
- Communicative and informative.
- Kind, compassionate and helpful.
- Courteous, respectful, polite.
- Prompt, efficient, responsive.
- Clean and neat (facilities and personnel).

Techniques for Assessing Loyalty

MacStravic also says that although most physicians have not been trained in customer service, they have some idea as to whether the patients are satisfied and loyal and why. As a group, however, physicians tend to overestimate patient satisfaction. The more they focus on the clinical side, the more likely doctors will miss something on the personal service side. It may be a good idea for doctors in a group or network setting to conduct self-audits during the same time period patients are questioned on satisfaction and loyalty issues. This self-audit of patient satisfaction should be accurate and honest. Doctors should imagine themselves as the patient and answer questions that include:

- Are there any complaints from patients about the staff's attitude and behavior, and is it clear to whom they can report these concerns? Is there a system for follow up?
- Do patients view physicians and staff as friendly and hospitable toward them and their families?
- Does the practice periodically examine all systems that greatly affect patient satisfaction and try to improve them?
- Have we looked at the amenities we offer to see whether or how they should be changed for patient comfort?
- Are there systems in place that regularly assess the satisfaction level of patients?
- Do we offer conveniences such as ease-of-payment, extended office hours, or parking facilities?
- Is attendance at training programs to improve personal service skills encouraged?

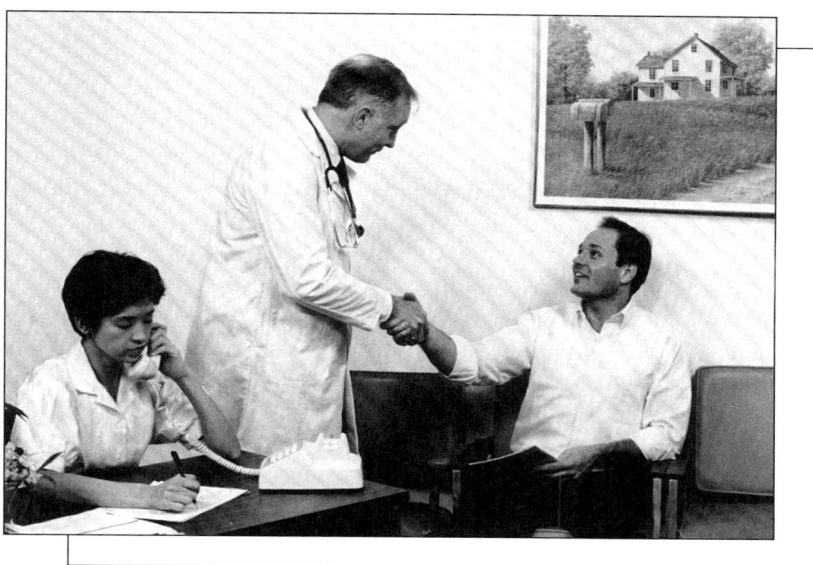

The self-audit makes it possible for a practice to keep reviewing its strengths, identify and improve its weaknesses and, over a period of time, create a service-oriented culture where patients' needs are met.

Some of the same techniques used when surveying patients on their satisfaction with individual physician visits can be applied to promote satisfaction with and commitment to the practice as a whole. Patients can be asked questions like:

- In your experience with the professionals (doctors, staff) of this practice, what have you liked? What have you disliked?

- Are there specific instances when you wished things were handled differently? By the doctor? By the staff?

- Could the office environment be improved?

- Are there systems (phone, scheduling appointments, billing) you would like to see improved?

- Are you provided with clear and concise information?

- How can this practice better serve you in the future?

- Would you recommend this practice to family or friends?

With regular self-audits and patient surveys in place, physicians and their staffs will become more sensitive to the role satisfaction plays in patient retention and loyalty.

Putting Results to Work

Once the results of self-audits are compiled and patient input has been tabulated, the first order of business is to make the most obvious and easiest changes that are called for. A letter to patients should follow as soon as possible. It should indicate:

- Appreciation for patient participation in the process of change.
- Announcement of immediate changes that have resulted.
- Future plans based on information gathered.
- Instructions for submitting further suggestions.
- Improving Staff Attitudes and Behavior

Today's physicians don't have a lot of time to attend to staff management. Hiring an office manager as part of the team could be the solution. This doesn't mean that physicians abdicate their role in decision-making. They should try to meet weekly with the office manager to ferret out staff problems and make sure all systems are running smoothly.

Consider the following scenario:

A practice has adopted the philosophy—"patients come first"—mentioned in the last chapter. Long-term employees have been informed that improving interpersonal skills will be a critical indicator of job success. The interview process for potential new employees includes discussion of the subject.

The physicians have determined that skills such as treating patients with courtesy, empathy and helpfulness, and dealing with angry people and their complaints in a calm and caring manner, are important for patient satisfaction. They also have formulated these strategies to meet their goal:

- Each level of staff is provided with information on interpersonal skill development appropriate for the job.
- There is a yearly budget that includes in-house training and tuition reimbursement for the enhancement of interpersonal skills.
- Staff members are reviewed every six months, complimented on their strengths, and encouraged to improve on their weaknesses.
- Service is rewarded either monetarily, by granting extra paid time off, or with a special gift.

In this busy practice, all-staff meetings are held every six months, prior to individual formal reviews. Specific interpersonal skills are discussed at each meeting, and staff is asked to fill out self-audit forms answering such questions as:

- Are you challenged by trying to solve an angry patient's complaint?
- Do you listen attentively to what the patient says?
- Do you answer in a calm and collected way?
- What are some ways that you solve problems with a dissatisfied patient?

Staff is encouraged to write a brief but definitive account in answer to each question. The self-audit becomes a speaking point to address during the employee review process.

Does Everybody Need Training?

According to *Patient Satisfaction: A Guide to Practice Management*, many staff members feel they already know how to be nice to patients. But the medical environment has many challenges—"handling complaints without defensiveness, calming an upset patient, dealing with angry people, easing a long wait, listening actively, and communicating disturbing information"—that require multifaceted skills. That's why it's necessary for physicians to set standards that meet their goals for patient satisfaction and to require that staff work towards this objective.

The book lists these training opportunities to strengthen staff skills:

Books and Other Print Resources. Going on-line (in the office, at home, or using the public library) is the best way to find sources for self-help and how-to books and articles on improving interpersonal skills. While it does not always provide the complete text, the Internet lists publishing sources and tells how to access information. It is also a good way to find out about available curriculum, including video and audio tapes, programmed instruction materials, and training designs.

Commercially Available Programs. Investigate one, two, or three-day training programs available nationwide and advertised on the Internet or in newspapers, medical journals, and professional association newsletters. Some of the programs are directed explicitly toward health care personnel; others are courses on customer relations for employees of any company in the service business.

In-House Training. Local hospitals, independent training providers, or universities are excellent sources of in-house training designed to meet specific needs. Once a practice has identified patient satisfaction goals, these in-house programs will teach the necessary interpersonal skills.

One-on-One Training. Giving staff members who excel in interpersonal skills mentoring or coaching responsibilities for others on staff adds dimension to their jobs and can be a very rewarding experience for them. Those who require attention benefit from knowing that their "trainers" have encountered the exact same situations and experienced the same frustrations, and so they respect their abilities and skills.

Staff Meetings. A staff meeting can be the perfect environment for improving behavior toward patients, building awareness, and creating the team spirit necessary to reach practice goals. To make this time meaningful and purposeful, the meeting must be well planned. For instance, if patient interaction is the focus, formats should encourage staff to offer problem-solving ideas and act out problem-solving behaviors.

Physicians should periodically ask themselves how their staff is doing. Are patients being treated with dignity? Have there been any complaints about interactions with patients' families? If patients are leaving for another doctor, what are the reasons?

If the answers to any of these questions raise doubts about staff behavior, then any amount of time and money invested in developing interpersonal skills will be well spent.

Physician Education

An article by Lewis Owen Amack, appearing on the Internet's *Lawinfo Forum*, reveals that it is only in the past 15 years that some medical education programs have adopted the biopsychosocial approach, integrating biomedical knowledge with interpersonal and interviewing skills.

The advantages to this approach to medical education are:

- Students focus on the full set of skills needed to be an effective healer.

- They learn to appreciate patients not just in terms of medical dysfunction, but also as human beings, each with a unique personal history and values.

- It leads to a mutually beneficial relationship between physicians and patients.

Goals in developing interpersonal skills for medical students include:

- Creating more productive and positive relations with patients.

- Reducing the liability of malpractice suits.

- Making the clinical experience more gratifying.

- Increasing patient adherence to their treatments.

Current teaching methods include simulating patients in role-play and video-taping practice interviews in small-group sessions where both verbal and non-verbal communications are emphasized.

Many authorities still point to the lack of interpersonal skills taught in medical schools as a drawback. An August 13, 1997, article appearing in the *Journal of the American Medical Association* agrees. Entitled, "Calibrating the physician: personal awareness and effective patient care," the article advocates the recognition of emotional resources and experiences as key to improving the physician-patient relationship. Unrecognized feelings and behaviors may get in the way of physician-patient communication; limit the physician's ability to feel empathy for patients; interfere with meaningful exchanges on hard-to-discuss topics such as sexuality, aging, death and dying; and encourage under- or over-involvement with patients. The authors suggest some topics and questions that should be addressed as part of:

Personal Awareness Curriculum:

Gender Issues
Do I respond differently to male and female patients? Male and female colleagues?

Anger, Conflict
What types of patients or work situations anger me?

Difficult Patients
Are personal biases interfering with how I deal with my patients?

Caring for Dying Patients
How have my own personal losses affected my ability to care for dying patients?

Balancing Personal and Professional Life
What would be the ideal balance of work, play, family, and personal growth?

Preventing and Managing Stress/Burnout/Impairment
Have I ever experienced or am I now experiencing work overload, personal problems, or anxiety due to patients' suffering?

Motivating Physicians

Interpersonal training programs for physicians abound. Most of them are based on the assumptions that:

- Today's patients judge physicians not only on quality of care, but their interpersonal skills as well.

- There are behaviors and techniques that will improve physician-patient relations and, if physicians are motivated, they can be learned.

How can the motivated physician change? According to the authors of *Patient Satisfaction: A Guide to Practice Enhancement*, "First of all, physicians need to know what they already do behaviorally and its effects on or consequences for patient satisfaction. This calls for feedback." They go on to say that patient surveys are one way to receive feedback. But the other, more powerful way, is to have knowledgeable people guide physicians by giving them choices and alternatives for interacting with patients.

"Can't get no (patient) satisfaction? Try charm school," states an article in the October 14, 1996, *Medical Economic Journal*. It reports on in-house training programs for doctors provided by Kaiser Permanente. Before Kaiser's Northern California group began offering patient relations courses to physicians, 52 percent of physicians said that more than 10 percent of their patient visits were frustrating. After completing the course, only 34 percent felt that way. Some of the twelve Kaiser Permanente regions provide one-day workshops and individual coaching as needed; others focus on ongoing training.

Physician communication skills and improved physician-patient relations are teachable, learnable skills. By offering more opportunities to improve interpersonal skills, and by increasing the number of medical schools that offer these skills to their students, we will see a greater gratification for both physicians and patients in their relationship.

Physicians who recognize a deficit when it comes to their interpersonal skills have many courses to choose from. These are just some of the many seminar and workshop providers:

The Bayer Institute For Health Care Communication
488 Wheelers Farms Road, Milford, CT 06460
800-800-5907

Northwest Center for Physician-Patient Communication
Foundation for Medical Excellence
4000 Kruse Way Place, Building 2, Suite 100, Lake Oswego, OR 97035
503-636-2234

American College of Physician Executives
4890 W Kennedy Boulevard, Suite 200, Tampa, FL 33609-2575
818-287-2000

Kaset International
8875 Hidden River Parkway, Tampa, FL 33637
813-977-8875

Bibliography

Amack LO. Enhancing physician-patient rapport. *Lawinfo Forum*. November 8, 1995.

Susan Keane Baker, "Ten Steps to Better Service," *American Medical News*, February 24, 1997.

Bendall D, Powers TL. Cultivating loyal patients. *Journal of Health Care Marketing*. Winter 1995.

"Beware of Online Info," *Chicago Tribune*, June 11, 1998.

"Communication Skills Cut Malpractice Risk," Society for the Advancement of Education. *USA Today*, October 1997.

"Consumer Complaint Department," *People's Medical Society, Inc.* (newsletter), April 1997.

Sherilyn L. Cormier, William H. Cormier, and Roland J. Weisser Jr. *Interviewing and Helping Skills for Health Care Professionals.* Boston: Jones and Bartlett Publishers, Inc., 1986.

Gianakos D. Empathy revisited. *Archives of Internal Medicine*. January 22, 1996.

Susan Gilbert, "Forget About Bedside Manners, Some Doctors Have No Manners," *New York Times,* December 23, 1997.

Grandinetti D. Can't get no (patient) satisfaction? Try charm school. *Medical Economics*. October 14, 1996.

Regina E. Herzlinger. *Market-Driven Health Care.* Reading, Mass.:Addison-Wesley Publishing Company, Inc., 1997.

"Hey Doc, Let's Talk!" *People's Medical Society, Inc.* (newsletter), August 1997.

Is good communication synonymous with high patient satisfaction? *The Back Letter,* Skol Corporation, February 1996.

Wendy Leebov, Michael Vergare, MD, and Gail Scott, MA. *Patient Satisfaction: A Guide to Practice Management.* Oradell, NJ: Medical Economics Books, 1990.

MacStravic R. Scott. *Beyond Patient Satisfaction*. Chicago:American College of Healthcare Executives; 1991.

MacStravic RS. Patient loyalty to physicians. *Journal of Health Care Marketing*, Winter 1994.

Leonard J Marcus and Barry C Dorn, "Negotiating an Effective Physician-Patient Relationship," *American Medical News*, July 7, 1997.

Mummalaneni V, Gopalakrishna P. Mediators vs. moderators of patient satisfaction. *Journal of Health Care Marketing*, Winter 1995.

Novack DH, Suchman AL, Clark W, Epstein RM, Najberg E, Kaplan C. *Calibrating the physician: personal awareness and effective patient care.* American Medical Association; *JAMA.* 1997;278:502-509.

Jane Oliva, "How to Remove Wedges Between Patients, Doctors,*"American Medical News*, May 13, 1996.

"A Survey of the Patient-Physician Relationship in America," conducted by Yankelovich Partners, Pfizer Medical Humanities Initiative, April 1998.

Ken Terry. *How To Get the Best Reading Of Patient Satisfaction.* Medical Economics Publishing; July 15, 1996.

Richard K. Thomas. *Health Care Consumers in the 1990s.* Ithaca, New York: American Demographics Books, 1993.

David Zimmerman, Peggy Zimmerman, and Charles Lund. *The Healthcare Customer Service Revolution.* Burr Ridge, Ill.: Irwin Professional Publishing, 1996.

Abigail Zuger, "When the Doctor and Patient Need Couple's Therapy," *New York Times*, March 31, 1998.